DISCLAIMER

This information is not intended as a substitute for professional medical advice, emergency treatment or formal first-aid training.

Don't use this information to diagnose or develop treatment plan for a health problem or disease without consulting a qualified health care provider.

If you are in a life threatening or emergency medical situation, please seek medical assistance immediately

BRAIN

ANEURYSM

Surviving Aneurysm

CHARLES MORTON

Contents

CHAPTER ONE

DEFINITION

A mind aneurysm is a lump or expanding in a vein in the cerebrum. It frequently seems as though a berry holding tight a stem.

A mind aneurysm can break or burst, causing seeping into the cerebrum (hemorrhagic stroke). Frequently a burst mind aneurysm happens in the space between the cerebrum and the dainty tissues covering the mind. This sort of hemorrhagic stroke is known as a subarachnoid drain.

A burst aneurysm rapidly gets perilous and requires brief clinical treatment.

Most cerebrum aneurysms, nonetheless, don't crack, make medical issues or cause indications. Such aneurysms are regularly recognized during tests for different conditions.

Treatment for an unruptured mind aneurysm might be fitting at times and may forestall a break later on.

Aneurysm rupture: The primary symptom of a ruptured aneurysm is a severe headache. This headache is frequently described as the "worst headache" ever felt.

The following are common signs and symptoms of a ruptured aneurysm:

• A severe headache that appears out of nowhere.

• Vomiting and nausea

- A stiff neck

- Double or blurred vision

- Light sensitivity

- Convulsions

- A droopy eyelid

- Consciousness loss

- Perplexity

Aneurysm that is 'leaking'

An aneurysm may leak a small amount of blood in some cases. This leaking (sentinel bleed) may only result in:

• A severe headache that appears out of nowhere.

Leaking is almost always followed by a more severe rupture.

Aneurysm that has not ruptured

An unruptured brain aneurysm may not cause any symptoms, especially if it is small. A large unruptured aneurysm, on the other hand, may press on brain tissues and nerves, potentially causing:

• Eye pain (both above and behind the eye)

• A pupil that is dilated

• Vision change or double vision

• Facial numbness, weakness, or paralysis on one side

• A droopy eyelid

Seek immediate medical attention if you develop any of the following symptoms:

• A severe headache that appears out of nowhere.

Call 911 or your local emergency number if you are with someone who has a sudden, severe headache, loses consciousness, or has a seizure.

Aneurysms in the brain develop as a result of thinning artery walls. Because those sections of the vessel are weaker, aneurysms frequently form at forks or branches in arteries.

Aneurysms can occur anywhere in the brain, but they are most common in arteries near the brain's base.

CHAPTER TWO

RISK FACTORS OF BRAIN ANEURYSMS

A variety of factors can contribute to artery wall weakness and increase the risk of a brain aneurysm. Adults are more likely than children to have a brain aneurysm, and women are more likely than men to have one.

Some of these risk factors emerge gradually over time, while others are present at birth.

Factors of risk that emerge over time

These are some examples:

• Growing older

• Cigarette smoking

• Hypertension (high blood pressure) (hypertension)

• Atherosclerosis (hardening of the arteries) (arteriosclerosis)

• Substance abuse, particularly cocaine use

• A brain injury

• Excessive alcohol consumption

• Specific blood infections

• Lower estrogen levels following menopause

Risk factors that are present at birth

These are some examples:

• Inherited connective tissue disorders that weaken blood vessels, such as Ehlers-Danlos syndrome

• Polycystic kidney disease, an inherited condition that causes fluid-filled sacs in the kidneys and typically raises blood pressure.

• An abnormally narrow aorta, a large blood vessel that transports oxygen-rich blood from the heart to the body.

• Cerebral arteriovenous malformation, an abnormal connection between the brain's arteries and veins that disrupts the normal flow of blood between them.

• A first-degree relative, such as a parent, brother, or sister, who has a family history of brain aneurysm.

When a brain aneurysm ruptures, the bleeding is usually only a few seconds long. Blood can directly harm surrounding cells, and bleeding can harm or kill other cells. It also causes an increase in intracranial pressure.

If the pressure rises too high, the blood and oxygen supply to the brain may be disrupted, resulting in loss of consciousness or even death.

Following an aneurysm rupture, the following complications may occur:

• Rebreeding An aneurysm that has ruptured or leaked may bleed again. Rebreeding can harm brain cells even more.

Vasospasm is a condition in which the blood vessels constrict. Blood vessels in your brain may narrow erratically after a brain aneurysm ruptures (vasospasm). This condition can reduce blood flow to brain cells and cause additional cell damage and loss (ischemic stroke).

• Hydrocephalus is a condition in which the brain is flooded with water. When an aneurysm ruptures, causing bleeding in the space between the brain and surrounding tissue (subarachnoid hemorrhage), the blood can obstruct circulation of the fluid surrounding the brain and spinal cord (cerebrospinal fluid).

This condition can cause an excess of cerebrospinal fluid, which increases pressure on the brain and damages tissues (hydrocephalus).

• Hyponatremia is a condition in which there is a lack of sodium in the A ruptured brain aneurysm's subarachnoid hemorrhage can upset the sodium balance in the blood supply. This could be caused by damage to the hypothalamus, which is located near the base of the brain.

A drop in blood sodium levels can cause brain cell swelling and permanent damage.

CHAPTER THREE

Aneurysms in the brain are usually discovered after they have ruptured and become a medical emergency. A brain aneurysm, on the other hand, may be discovered after you've had head-imaging tests for another condition.

If the results of such tests indicate that you have a brain aneurysm, you should consult with a specialist in brain and nervous system disorders (neurologist or neurosurgeon).

To make the most of your time with your doctor, prepare a list of questions, such as:

• What do you know about the aneurysm's size and location?

• Do the imaging test results show how likely it is to rupture?

• At this time, what treatment do you recommend?

• How often will I need to have follow-up tests if we wait?

• What precautions can I take to reduce the risk of an aneurysm rupturing?

To help determine the best course of action, your neurologist or neurosurgeon may ask you the following questions:

• Do you use tobacco?

• How much alcohol do you consume?

• Do you use drugs for fun?

• Do you have high blood pressure, high cholesterol, or any other conditions that increase your risk of cardiovascular disease?

• Do you take your medications exactly as directed by your doctor?

• Do you have a family history of brain aneurysms?

CHAPTER FOUR

If you have a sudden, severe headache or other symptoms that could be caused by a ruptured aneurysm, you will be subjected to a test or series of tests to determine whether you have had bleeding into the space between your brain and surrounding tissues (subarachnoid hemorrhage) or another type of stroke.

If bleeding has occurred, your emergency care team will

determine whether it is the result of a ruptured aneurysm.

If you have symptoms of an unruptured brain aneurysm, such as pain behind the eye, changes in vision, or paralysis on one side of your face, you will most likely be subjected to the same tests.

Among the diagnostic tests are:

• Computed tomography (CT). A CT scan, which is a specialized X-ray exam, is usually the first test used to determine if you have brain bleeding. The test generates images of 2-D "slices" of the brain.

You may also be given a dye injection as part of this test, which makes it easier to see blood flow in the brain and may indicate the location of a ruptured aneurysm. CT angiography is the name given to this variant of the test.

• Cerebrospinal fluid analysis. There will almost certainly be red blood cells in the fluid surrounding your brain and spine if you have had a subarachnoid hemorrhage (cerebrospinal fluid).

If you have symptoms of a ruptured aneurysm but a CT scan shows no evidence of bleeding, your doctor will order a cerebrospinal fluid test.

A lumbar puncture, also known as a spinal tap, is a procedure that uses a needle to extract cerebrospinal fluid from your back.

• Magnetic resonance imaging (MRI). An MRI creates detailed images of the brain using a magnetic field and radio waves, either in 2-D slices or 3-D images.

An MRI that examines the arteries in great detail may detect the location of a ruptured aneurysm.

• A cerebral angiogram is a type of angiogram that looks at the blood vessels in the brain. Your doctor will insert a thin, flexible tube (catheter) into a large artery — usually in your groin — and thread it past your heart to the arteries in your brain during this procedure, also known as a cerebral arteriogram. A special dye injected into the catheter travels to the arteries in your brain.

A series of X-ray images can then reveal information about your arteries' conditions and the location of a ruptured aneurysm. This test is more invasive than others and is typically used when other diagnostic tests are insufficient.

Brain aneurysm screening

It is not generally recommended to use imaging tests to screen for unruptured brain aneurysms. However, you should talk to your doctor about the potential benefits of a screening test if you have:

• A parent or sibling with a ruptured brain aneurysm, especially if you have two such first-degree relatives with brain aneurysms.

• A congenital disorder that increases your chances of developing a brain aneurysm.

CHAPTER FIVE

DRUGS AND TREATMENTS

For a ruptured brain aneurysm, there are two common treatment options.

• Surgical clipping is a procedure that is used to close an aneurysm. To access the aneurysm, the neurosurgeon removes a section of your skull and locates the blood vessel that feeds the aneurysm. Then he or she places a tiny metal clip around the aneurysm's neck to stop blood flow to it.

Endovascular coiling is a less invasive alternative to surgical clipping. A hollow plastic tube (catheter) is inserted into an artery, usually in your groin, and threaded through your body to the aneurysm.

He or she then inserts a soft platinum wire through the catheter and into the aneurysm using a guide wire. The wire coils up inside the aneurysm, causing blood flow to be disrupted and clotting. Clotting effectively seals the aneurysm from the artery.

Both procedures are risky, especially if there is bleeding in the brain or a loss of blood flow to the brain. The endovascular coil is less invasive and may be initially safer, but it also has a higher risk of subsequent re-bleeding and may necessitate additional procedures.

New treatments for brain aneurysms, such as flow diverters, are now available. These may be especially useful in larger aneurysms that cannot be treated safely with other options.

Your neurosurgeon or interventional neuroradiologist will make a recommendation in collaboration with your neurologist based on the size, location, and overall appearance of the brain aneurysm, your ability to undergo a procedure, and other factors.

Other therapies

Other treatments for ruptured brain aneurysms are aimed at symptom relief and management of complications.

• To treat headache pain, pain relievers such as acetaminophen (Tylenol, among others) may be used.

• Calcium channel blockers prevent calcium from entering blood vessel wall cells. These medications may help to reduce the erratic narrowing of blood vessels (vasospasm) that can occur as a result of a ruptured aneurysm.

One of these medications, nimodipine , has been shown to reduce the risk of delayed brain injury caused by insufficient blood flow following a ruptured aneurysm subarachnoid hemorrhage.

• Interventions to prevent stroke due to insufficient blood flow include intravenous injections of a vasopressor, a drug that raises blood pressure to overcome the resistance of narrowed blood vessels.

Angioplasty is an alternative treatment for stroke prevention. A catheter is used to inflate a tiny balloon that expands a narrowed blood vessel in the brain during this procedure. A catheter can also be used to deliver a drug called a vasodilator to the brain, which causes blood vessels to dilate. Seizures caused by a ruptured aneurysm may be treated with anti-seizure medications. • Ventricular or lumbar draining catheters and shunt surgery can relieve pressure on the brain caused by excess cerebrospinal fluid (hydrocephalus) caused by a ruptured aneurysm. A catheter may be inserted into the fluid-filled spaces inside your brain (ventricles) or around your brain and spinal cord to drain the excess fluid into an external bag.

• Rehabilitative therapy. It may be necessary to introduce a shunt system, which consists of a flexible silicone rubber tube (shunt) and a valve that creates a drainage channel starting in your brain and ending in your abdominal cavity. Subarachnoid hemorrhage brain damage may necessitate physical, speech, and occupational therapy to relearn skills.

Unruptured brain aneurysm treatment

Endovascular coiling or surgical clipping can be used to seal off an unruptured brain aneurysm and help prevent future rupture. However, in some unruptured aneurysms, the procedures' known risks may outweigh the potential benefit.

A neurologist, working with a neurosurgeon or interventional neuroradiologist, can help you decide whether the treatment is right for you.

They would consider the following factors when making a

recommendation: • the size, location, and overall appearance of the aneurysm

• Your age and general health • A family history of ruptured aneurysms • Congenital conditions that increase the risk of aneurysm rupture

If you have high blood pressure, consult your doctor about treatment options. If you have a brain aneurysm, keeping your blood pressure under control may reduce your risk of rupture.

Furthermore, if you smoke cigarettes, speak with your provider about smoking cessation strategies, as cigarette smoking may be a risk factor for the formation, growth, and rupture of the aneurysm.

CHAPTER FIVE

If you have an unruptured brain aneurysm, you can reduce your risk of rupture by making the following lifestyle changes:

• Avoid smoking and using recreational drugs. If you smoke or use recreational drugs, speak with your doctor about quitting strategies or an appropriate treatment program.

• Maintain a healthy diet and exercise routine. Dietary and exercise changes can help lower blood pressure. Consult your doctor about making changes that are right for you.

• Keep caffeine to a minimum. Caffeine is a stimulant that can cause a spike in blood pressure.

• Avoid squeezing. Sudden, forceful, and sustained exertion, such as that required to lift heavy weights, can cause an increase in blood pressure.

THE END

Other Books by Author

1. http://getbook.at/THE-LUPUS-GUIDE

2. http://getbook.at/FLACCID-ACUTE-MYELITIS

3. http://getbook.at/SCHIZOPHRENIA

www.ingramcontent.com/pod-product-compliance
Lightning Source LLC
Chambersburg PA
CBHW061738250726
48657CB00002B/990